Enhancing Clinical Outcomes by Optimising the Therapeutic Relationship/Interaction

Duncan Lawler

- **Patient and Practitioner Influences on the Placebo Effect in Irritable Bowel Syndrome**
  John M Kelley, Anthony J Lembo, J Stuart Ablon, Joel J Villanueva, Lisa A Conboy, Ray Levy, Carl D Marci, Catherine Kerr, Irving Kirsch, Eric E Jacobson, Helen Riess and Ted J Kaptchuk
  Psychosom Med. 2009 September ; 71(7): 789. doi:10.1097/PSY.0b013e3181acee12

"There were significant differences between practitioners in outcomes, and this effect was twice as large as the effect attributable to treatment group assignment."

"Practitioners differed markedly in effectiveness despite standardized interactions"

Slide 1

PATIENT AND PRACTITIONER PLACEBO EFFECTS

Kelley JM, Lembo AJ, Ablon JS, Villanueva JJ, Conboy LA, Levy R, et al. Patient and practitioner influences on the placebo effect in irritable bowel syndrome. *Psychosom Med* 2009;71:789–97. PMID 19661195

Slide 2

Brinkhaus B, Witt CM, Jena S, et al. **Acupuncture in patients with allergic rhinitis: a pragmatic randomized trial.** Ann Allergy, Asthma Immunol 2008;101:535–43.

- " it seems that physician characteristics play a minor role in the effectiveness of acupuncture treatment, although this idea needs further investigation"

Slide 3

The Irritable Bowel Syndrome: long term prognosis and the physician-patient interaction.
Owens DM, Nelson DK, Talley NJ.
Ann Intern Med. 1995 Jan 15;122(2): 107-112

- "A positive physician-patient interaction may be related to reduced use of ambulatory health services by patients with IBS."

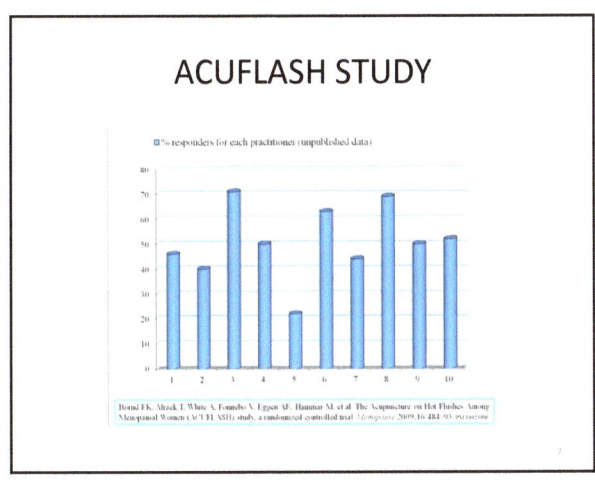

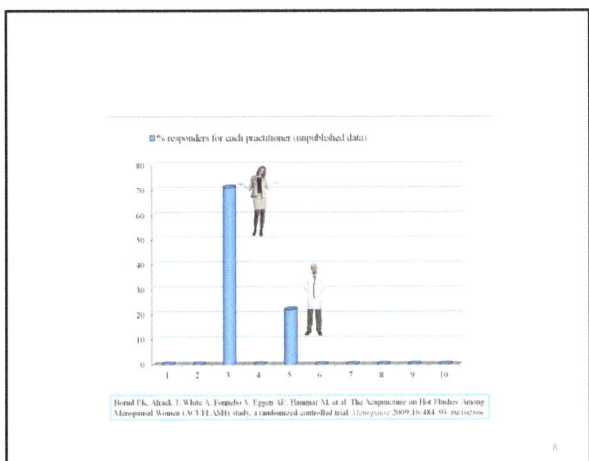

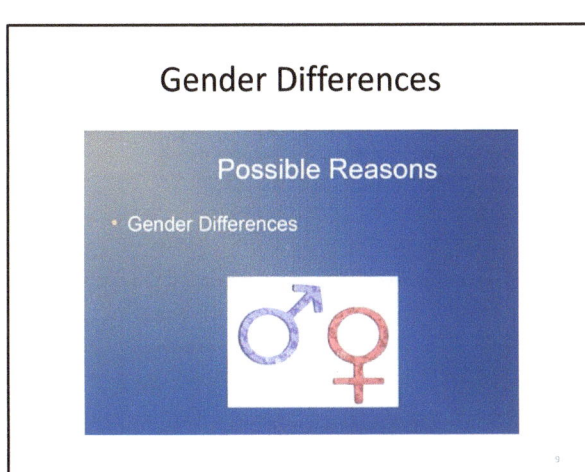

Gender Differences

Communication

Male · Female
Speech and language areas of the brain, Institute of Psychiatry, London, 2001.

This visual was created from brain scans of 50 men and women, showing the active areas of the brain (in black) that are used for speech and language.
It's a graphic image of men and women talking and communicating with each other.

The shaded areas are used for speech and language function. Women have a natural greater capacity for talking than men.

Differences

- Female 6,000 – 8000 spoken words per day
- Male 2,000 – 4000 spoken words per day

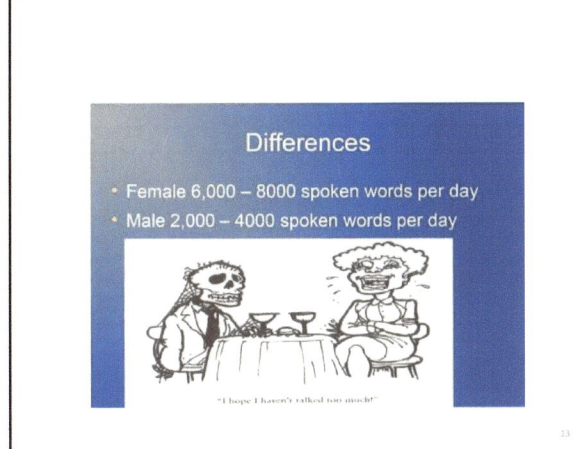

"I hope I haven't talked too much!"

13

Male Communication

Men use speech and language to communicate facts and data.

This is what's wrong

This is what I'm going to do

This is what I'm doing

This is what I've done

14

Male Brain

The male brain is configured for problem solving and to continually come up with solutions. 'Men are from Mars, Women are from Venus'

This approach is direct and effective for male patients. However as I discovered it's not so effective with females!

15

Female Communication

Female 'talk' is used as a form of reward and to bond with another person.

The dynamics of the therapeutic relationship can affect the outcome of treatments according to Kelley and Kaptchuck

16

A female brain is organised for multi-tracking. She can talk about several unrelated topics of conversation and uses five vocal tones to change the subject or emphasise points. Men can identify only three of those tones

17

Relationship

People relate to people similar to them. Dwoertzky 1994

The dynamics of the therapeutic relationship would potentially be compromised were a Male acupuncturist not to adapt his communication approach to females.

He would appear cold and disinterested which is untrue as he is just problem focussed and not person focussed

18

Also the Female acupuncturist perhaps may appear unfocussed to the male as he would have difficulty seeing the point of her talking.

ZONES

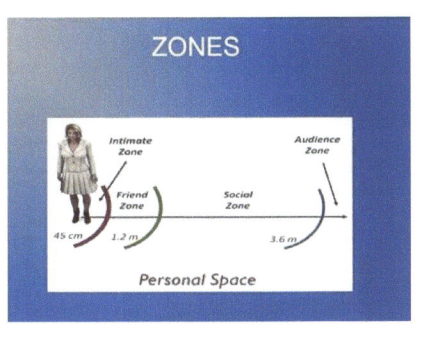

Personal Space

Intimate Zone: About 15 to 45 cm's (6 to 18 inches) this is the most important zone of them all as it is only reserved for a select few of people, this includes parents, love partners, children, family and very close friends, the proximity chosen by the person is also dependant on who it is.

Anyone who is not meant to be in the Intimate Zone and enters it will cause physiological changes (such as increased heart rate) in our body as we will feel threatened.

Hence the importance of establishing trust in the Therapeutic Relationship.

This anxiety is magnified when it is a member of the opposite sex.
(Morris 1977)

The amygdala is suspected of processing people's strong reactions to personal space violations since these are absent in those in which it is damaged and it is activated when people are physically close. (Kennedy et al 2009)

CCK

Anxious patients have raised levels of CCK (Cholecystokinin) and therefore are likely to experience more pain.

A relaxed patient will have lower levels of CCK and better results with acupuncture theoretically.
(White/Cummings/Filshie 2008)

White/Cummings and Filshie also state that it is important to prepare patients for acupuncture in ways that reduce anxiety, such as avoiding rush, providing adequate explanation, leaving opportunites for questions and discussion.

Perhaps in certain cases identifying the correct gender in the specific case may also reduce anxiety?

- **The Effect of Treatment Expectation on Drug Efficacy: Imaging the Analgesic Benefit of the Opioid Remifentanil**
  Ulrike Bingel, Vishvarani Wanigasekera, Katja Wiech, Roisin Ni Mhuircheataigh, Micahel C. Lee, Markus Ploner, Irene Tracey.
  Science Translational Medicine 70ra 14 (2011)

"Positive treatment expectancy substantially enhanced (doubled) the analgesic benefit of remifentanil. In contrast, negative treatment expectancy abolished remifentanil analgesia."

"The positive expectancy effects were associated with activity in the endogenous pain modulatory system, and the negative expectancy effects with activity in the hippocampus."

The Nocebo Response

The term "nocebo response" originally meant an unpredictable unintentional belief-generated injurious response to an inert procedure.

An example of nocebo effect would be someone who dies of fright after being bitten by a non-venomous snake.

28

The Nocebo Effect

The term "nocebo response" was coined in 1961 by Walter Kennedy.

Kennedy chose the Latin word *nocebo* ("I shall harm") because it was the opposite of the Latin word placebo ("I shall please"), and used it to denote the counterpart of the placebo response: namely, an "unpleasant" response to the application of real or sham treatment.

29

He insisted that a *nocebo reaction* was subject-centred, and he was emphatic that the term *nocebo reaction* specifically referred to "a quality inherent in the patient rather than in the remedy"

30

Kennedy was speaking of an outcome that had been totally generated by a subject's *negative expectation* of a treatment; which was the exact counterpart of a *placebo response* that would have been generated by a subject's *positive expectation*.

It is therefore plausible that where one gender may have greater rates of success with specific genders with certain conditions and this partly can be due to the placebo effect, the opposite could occur with the incorrect gender and actually have a negative outcome as opposed to having no effect – the nocebo effect. BUT WHY?

- BECAUSE OF THE INCREASE in LEVELS OF ANXIETY – POSSIBLY ELEVATED LEVELS OF CCK - NOCEBO

Reducing Anxiety

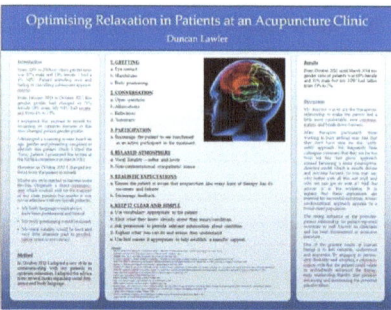

Introduction

From 2001 to 2008 my client gender ratio was 87% male and 13% female. I had a 4% NFU. (Patient attending once and failing or cancelling subsequent appointments).

From January 2009 to October 2012 this gender profile had changed to 71% female 29% male. My NFU had increased from 4% to 23%.

I explained this increase to myself by focussing on common features of this now changed patient gender profile.

I developed a screening system based on age, gender and presenting complaint to identify this patient which I titled the 'Toxic' patient. I presented this lecture at the NFMA conference in March 2012.

However in October 2012 I changed my focus from the patient to myself.

> "Everyone thinks of changing the world but no one thinks of changing himself."
>
> Leo Tolstoy

Maybe my style needed to become more flexible. Originally a direct communicator which worked well for the majority of my male patients but maybe it was not as effective with my female patients.

- My body language would always have been professional and formal.
- My body positioning would be closed.
- My vocal tonality would be loud and very little attention paid to psychological space or eye contact.

Method

In October 2012 I adopted a new style in communicating with my patients to optimise relaxation. I adapted the advice from several books regarding social dynamics and body language.

1. GREETING
a. Eye contact
b. Handshake
c. Body positioning.

2. CONVERSATION
a. Open questions
b. Affirmations
c. Reflections
d. Summary.

3. PARTICIPATION
a. Encourage the patient to see him/herself as an active participant in the treatment.

4. RELAXED ATMOSPHERE
a. Vocal Tonality – softer and lower
b. Non-confrontational, sympathetic stance.

5. REALISTIC EXPECTATIONS
a. Ensure the patient is aware that acupuncture like every form of therapy has it's successes and failures
b. Encourage feedback.

6. KEEP IT CLEAR AND SIMPLE
a. Use vocabulary appropriate to the patient
b. Elicit what they know already about their injury/condition
c. Ask permission to provide relevant information about condition
d. Explain what you can do and ensure they understand
e. Use first names if appropriate to help establish a friendly rapport.

40

Results

From October 2012 until March 2014 my gender ratio of patients was 69% female and 31% male but my NFU had fallen from 23% to 7%.

41

My objective was to use the therapeutic relationship to make the person feel a little more comfortable, ease communication, and break down barriers.

Many therapists particularly those working in busy settings may feel that they don't have time for this 'softly softly' approach. We frequently hear colleagues comment that they are far too busy for this 'kid glove' approach instead favouring a more prescriptive, directive model which is results driven and outcome focused. So you may say why bother with all this soft stuff and why not just get on with it? Well the answer is in the evidence. It is argued that these aspirations are essential for successful outcomes. A non-confrontational approach appeals to a broad client population.

42

The strong influence of the provider-patient relationship on patient-reported outcomes is well known to clinicians and has been documented in extensive literature.

One of the greatest needs of human beings is to feel valuable, understood and important. By engaging in personality flexibility and adopting a communication style that the patient could relate to undoubtedly enhanced the therapeutic relationship thereby also possibly enhancing and maximising the potential placebo effect.

- **Patient and Practitioner Influences on the Placebo Effect in Irritable Bowel Syndrome**
  John M Kelley, Anthony J Lembo, J Stuart Ablon, Joel J Villanueva, Lisa A Conboy, Ray Levy, Carl D Marci, Catherine Kerr, Irving Kirsch, Eric E Jacobson, Helen Riess and Ted J Kaptchuk
  Psychosom Med. 2009 September ; 71(7): 789. doi:10.1097/PSY.0b013e3181acee12

"There were significant differences between practitioners in outcomes, and this effect was twice as large as the effect attributable to treatment group assignment."

"Practitioners differed markedly in effectiveness despite standardized interactions"

ACUFLASH

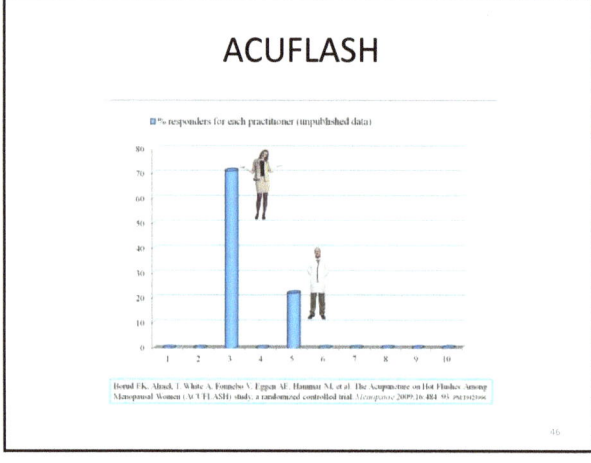

Berild Ek, Alraek, J. White A, Fonnebo V, Eggan AE, Hammar M, et al. The Acupuncture on Hot Flashes Among Menopausal Women (ACUFLASH) study, a randomized controlled trial. Menopause 2009;16:484-93.

LIKEABILITY & EMPATHY

- 5 PILLARS of LIKEABILITY
- 8 ELEMENTS OF EMPATHY
- TRIAD OF TOXICITY

---

5 Pillars of Likeability

1. EYE CONTACT

_____

_____

_____

_____

_____

_____

_____

2. BODY LANGUAGE

_____

_____

_____

_____

_____

_____

_____

3. Psychological Space

_____

_____

_____

_____

_____

_____

_____

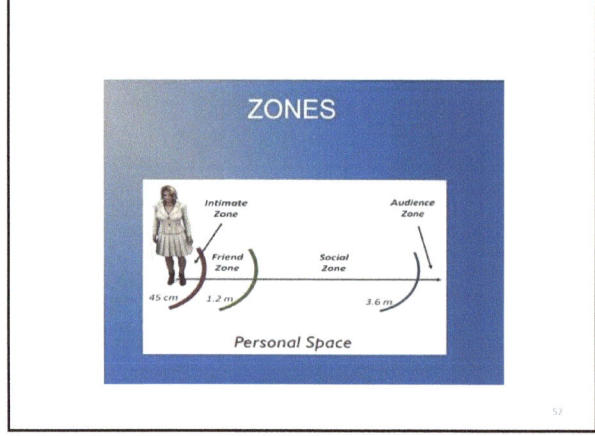

Intimate Zone: About 15 to 45 cm's (6 to 18 inches) this is the most important zone of them all as it is only reserved for a select few of people, this includes parents, love partners, children, family and very close friends, the proximity chosen by the person is also dependant on who it is.

Friend Zone: About 45 cms to 1.2 meters (18 to 46 inches) this is the distance we reserve for social gatherings such as parties, friendly interactions etc

Social Zone: About 1.2 to 3.5 meters (4 to 12 feet) this zoning is reserved for strangers we just met, acquaintances and anyone we interact with that we haven't established a relationship with.

Audience Zone: Anything over 3.5 meters (12 feet) is used to address an audience or large group of people.

4. Touch

5. Vocal Tonality

1. Slower and Lower
2. Remember Name and info and use it
3. NOTHING NEGATIVE e.g. never what's wrong etc.

---

5 Pillars of Likeability
1. Eye contact:
Look in to their left eye.
Concentrate on noticing their eye colour.

2. Body language:
Lean towards person from the left side.
Shoulders pointing towards them.
Feet pointing away.

3. Psychological Space:
Just enough space that if
You reached out you could
Hold their elbow

4. Touch:
When shaking hands
Let them release first

5. Vocal:
Use their name as much as you can
Speak lower and slower

Duncan Lawler

DEMO

8 Elements of Empathy

---

8 Elements of Empathy

1. Behavioural Default
2. Communication Style
3. Motivational Influence
4. Sensory Preference
5. Personality Type
6. Gender Role
7. Birth Order
8. Age

Duncan Lawler

---

1. Behavioural Default

Behaviour:

6. Supplicative
7. Combative
8. Competitive
9. Co-operative

64

---

2. Communication Style

Communication Style

1. Indirect & People focussed
2. Indirect & Task oriented
3. Direct & Task oriented
4. Direct & People focussed

66

3. Motivational Influence

Motivational Influence

6. External Accountability
7. Present Desire
8. Reasons
9. Outer & Inner Expectations

68

4. Sensory Preference

Sensory Preference

1. Visual
2. Auditory
3. Kinaesthetic

PEOPLE RELATE TO THOSE SIMILAR TO THEM. DWOERTSKY

Everybody has a primary sense that they use to perceive the world. Some people respond to the world and make their decisions based mostly on how things look, others by how things sound and others by physical sensation or how they feel

---

In the 1970's Richard Bandler and John Grinder, the founders of Neuro-Linguistic Programming, noticed in their early work with clients that people could be roughly divided into three types, depending on how they filtered the world through their senses. They called these types, VISUAL, AUDITORY and KINESTHETIC

No one is totally Visual, Auditory or 100% Kinesthetic. We are a mixture of all three but in every person, one of these systems (rather like left or right handedness) dominates the other two.

Studies have shown that as many as 55% of all people are motivated primarily by what they see, 15% by what they hear and 30% by physical

VISUAL TALK
How do you see yourself?
I see what you're saying.
He's such a colourful character.
A sight for sore eyes.
We are a company with a vision

AUDITORY TALK
Sounds Familiar
Tell me more
Let me tell you.
These colours are really loud
I didn't like his tone of voice

Kinesthetic Talk

Get over it.

Hang in there.

I can't put my finger on it.

Let's sort things out.

I'm not following you.

---

5. Personality Type

Personality Types:
6. Helper
7. Fighter
8. Doer
9. Everything

Personality Type:

The Helper:
Oestrogen
Doodles: Heart Flowers Faces Animals
Foods: Salads, Fruits, Veg
Sport: Yoga, Walking, Pilates

79

Fighter
Testosterone
Doodles: Squares Triangles Arrows
Food: Beef Chicken Beans Orange juice
Sports: Tennis Weights

80

The Doer
Dopamine

Doodles: Active Open
Food: Spicy Sweet
Sports: Sailing Rock Climbing

81

The Everything
Serotonin
Doodles: Repetitive Lines/ Grids
Food: Rice Potatoes Pasta
Bread Cereal Dairy Poultry Nuts
Sports: Social – Golf and Team sports

6. Gender Role

Gender Role

Male – Aggressive/Dominant

Female – Passive/Submissive

7. Birth Order

Birth Order

1. Only Child
2. Oldest Child
3. Middle Child
4. Youngest

Only Child

Leader
Self Control
Demanding
Self-Absorbed
Dependable
Private

Oldest

Leader
People Pleasers
High achiever
Organised and prompt
Controlling
Nurturing

Middle

Flexible
Easy going
Independent
Generous
Competitive
Possible victim complex

Youngest

Risk taker
Creative
Competitive
Inferiority Complex
Charming
Idealistic

8. Age

AGE:

1. UP TO 18
2. EARLY 20'S
3. 20'S
4. 30'S
5. EARLY 40'S
6. 40'S
7. 50'S and beyond

Up to 18:

1. Want to leave home
2. Break ties with their parents
3. Become their own person.

Early 20's

1. Start to discover who they really are.
2. Attracted to fads.

94

20's

1. Develop professionally
2. Influenced by mentors
3. Read more books
4. Education
5. Personal growth

95

30's

1. New vitality
2. Want to get out of rut
3. Ready for change
4. Possibly change career
5. Embark on new adventures

96

Mid 30's

1. Settle down
2. Feel as if time is running out on their goals.

Early 40's

1. Restless
2. Re-assessment and change especially if goals not met.

40's

1. Not the person they used to be
2. Stability
3. Give up on dreams when younger
4. Resignation

50's and beyond

1. Emotional time
2. Sullen/Depressed
3. Emerge strong, confident outspoken and secure
4. No nonsense approach to life

8 Elements of Empathy

1. Behavioural Default
2. Communication Style
3. Motivational Influence
4. Sensory Preference
5. Personality Type
6. Gender Role
7. Birth Order
8. Age

Duncan Lawler

An exaggerated extreme version

DEMO

4 FEATURES OF FASCINATING

1. Confidence:
Confidence is NOT "They will like me."
Confidence is "I'll be fine if they don't."

2. Humour:
Laugh at yourself.
Do not take yourself too seriously,
no one else does.

3. Edge:
Always be you:
When you smooth out your edges
to please others – you become
someone else others want you to be.

4. Detached:
Expect nothing
Accept everything
Judge nobody.

DUNCAN LAWLER

TRIAD OF TOXICITY

HANDLING NEGATIVE EMOTIONS
DEALING WITH EMOTIONAL FATIGUE

IDENITFYING THE EMOTION

1. HURT
2. ANGER
3. REGRET

Large-scale brain networks emerge from dynamic processing of musical timbre, key and rhythm.

Vinoo Alluri, Petri Toiviainen, Iiro P. Jääskeläinen, Enrico Glerean, Mikko Sams, Elvira Brattico. NeuroImage, 2011; DOI: 10.1016/j.neuroimage.2011.11.019

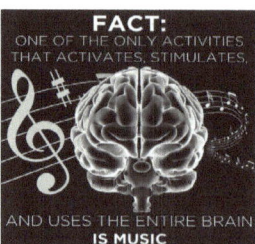

EFT

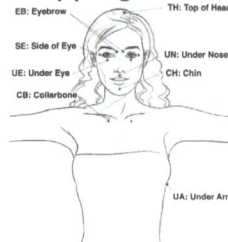

- **The efficacy of acupoint stimulation in the treatment of psychological distress: A meta-analysis.**
  Gilomen SA, Lee CW.
  J Behav Ther Exp Psychiatry. 2015 Sep;48:140-8

Emotional Freedom Techniques (EFT) is a type of therapy involving the stimulation of acupuncture points while using a spoken affirmation to target a psychological issue. The aim of this meta-analysis was to examine the effect of EFT, particular acupoint stimulation, in the treatment of psychological distress.

109

A moderate effect size and significantly high heterogeneity across studies was found using a random effects model indicating that EFT, even after removing outliers, **appears to produce an effect.** The analysis involved 12 studies comparing EFT with waitlist controls, 5 with adjuncts and only 1 comparison with an alternate treatment.

110

TRIAD OF TOXICITY

1. REGRET
2. ANGER
3. HURT

Duncan Lawler

111

IF IT ALL GOES WRONG

1. We are more vulnerable when we employ this system to being hurt.
2. What people say or do has rarely anything to do with us.
3. But we still get hurt , fall to pieces, Getting up
4. Reaching for ropes.

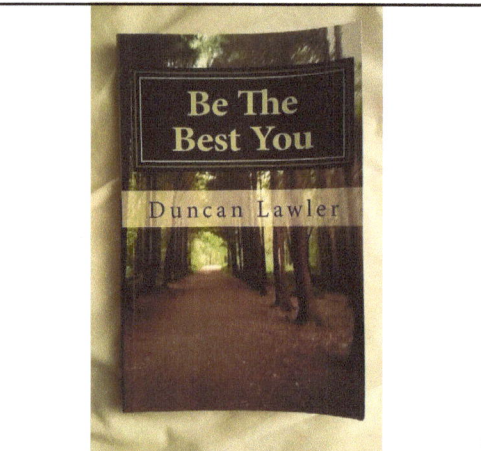